In the Event of Full Disclosure

In the Event of Full Disclosure

Poems by Cynthia Atkins

CW Books

Andrew —

So nice to
talk shop and
hope the words
find the place
on the page
for you.

Best

Published by CW Books
P.O. Box 541106
Cincinnati, OH 45254-1106

ISBN: 9781625490339
LCCN: 2013942730

Poetry Editor: Kevin Walzer
Business Editor: Lori Jareo

Visit us on the web at www.readcwbooks.com

Cover art and jacket design: "Mean Reds" by
          Christine Drake
Author photo: Julie Rivera Photography

For my siblings, Marla, Susan and Michael—

Under the seams runs the pain.

—Anne Carson

Grateful acknowledgment is made to the editors of the following publications who first published these poems:

Alaska Quarterly Review: "Montage Obscura," "Table"
Berkeley Poetry Review: "Closet"
Big City Lit: "Face Book," "Rumors Fly," "Diminution"
Bluestem Review: "In Plain Sight"
The Broome Review: "Letter to Metaphor"
Caketrain: "Family Therapy (III)"
Chelsea: "Terror in the Streets"
Clementine Magazine: "Divided We Stand," "Unreliable Narrator"
Comstock Review: "Frankenstein Meets Francis Bacon"
Del Sol Review: "Dear Reader," "Hillsides," "You Should Question"
descant: "Vacuum"
Eclipse: "You Know You're Alone"
The Florida Review: "Family Therapy (I)," "Family Therapy (II)," "Voices"
Good Foot: "Birth Right"
Harpur Palate: "Family Therapy (IV)"
Hawai'i Review: "When Homer Roams"
In Other Words: Merida: "Picture This," "Crickets," "Vacation"
Inertia Magazine: "Without A Visible Sign"
The Journal: "As Seen From Above"
Kalliope: "What the Blind See"
Le Zaporogue: "Disclosure"
Main Street Rag: "Country Mouse, City Mouse," "Vessels"
North American Review: "Elegy for a Scarecrow"
Open Window 5: "In a Parallel Universe"
Pearl: "Liturgy"
The Same: "Caribbean Fishing"
Saranac Review: "Rooms"
Sou'wester: "Zig-Zag"

Acknowledgments (continued)

Spiral Bridge: "Holes"
Street Light: "Etude for the Asking"
Tampa Review: "Shelf-Life"
Thema: "And So The Joke Goes"
Thrush: "TV"
Valparaiso Review: "Google Me"
Zocalo Public Square: "Nest"

The poems listed below also appeared in the following publications:

Askew: "In Plain Sight"
Canary: A Literary Journal of the Environmental Crisis: "When Homer Roams"
Cold Mountain Review: "Elegy for a Scarecrow"
Cultural Weekly: "Letter to Metaphor," "In Plain Sight," "Without a Visible Sign"
In Quire: "In Plain Sight"
Redux: "Liturgy"

Anthologies and Websites:

"In The Black/In The Red: Poems about Profit and Loss" (edited by Gloria Vando and Philip Miller)

"In Plain Sight" also appeared on the blog: *In Quire*

"Zig-Zag" and "Terror In The Streets" also appeared in *Juice Press* — http://juice-press.com/poetry2007/atkins/atkins.html

"Bernadette in Arches" with thanks and love to Jodi Nathenson

"Montage Obscura" with heartfelt thanks to Margaret Carroll, Bridget Kelley-Dearing, Mirabai McCleod for giving such time and love to my son, Eli

"Hillsides," with thanks to Daphne Raz for giving of her time and dedication

"In A Parallel Universe" inspired my writer friend, Seb Doubinsky

"Table" in honor of my amazing sister, Marla Snyder

"Foundry" written with love to my heroic sister, Susan Jacobs

"Birthright" for my one-of-a-kind son, Eli Welch

"You Should Question," a birthday poem for Duncan Richter

"Family Therapy V," in loving memory of my grandparents, Morris and Ida Wolf, and in honor of my mother, Barbara Wolf Mills

I want to express my heartfelt gratitude and appreciation to friends and family who have supported me with so much love, to colleagues and students, who keep me on my toes. I am grateful to the editors of journals that have sustained and nurtured these poems with much care and respect, and in the company of so many I admire. It has meant so much to me to have the love and support of my community: Rockbridge County, Chicago, friends near and far on my 'Facebook neighborhood,' that have graced my world with 'global' love and support.

To Phillip: friend, editor and love, for all of that and so much more

I was humbled by the grace of my readers: Jehanne Dubrow, Seb Doubinsky, Richard Tillinghast, and Lee Upton, who gave of their time and vision in agreeing to read the manuscript.

Heartfelt appreciation to Christine Drake, for lending her artwork, "Mean Reds" and her expert eye for the jacket design. I could not have done 'book one' or 'book two' without my right arm, Linda Morrison, who has edited and typed this book with so much loving care.

Thank you to Kevin Walzer and Lori Jareo for the production and the publication of this book.

Table of Contents

Part I

There's no vocabulary for love within a family, love that's lived in, but not looked at, love within the light of which all else is seen, the love within which all other love finds speech. This love is silent.

—T.S. Eliot

Liturgy

Because the trees grew
into paper for words to write
down what there are no words for.
Because it wants to size you up
and then compels you to confess.
Because it likes to breathe up
against you on the couch,
but will never commit to meals
or absolutes. Because it has no
understanding and no excuse,
and it dares the understudy
not to show up. Because you need
to get out of the weather, where
too many secrets are revealed
in the rain. Because it knows
you need to explain, even when
your hands are clean.
Because it told you
to spit out your gum
when a taxicab is running.
Because years have proven
that each death leads to song.
Because it knows the flowers
will be of no use—the words will dream
up the phlox. Because it will always
want and want to name what can't be named.
Because it knows you say one thing
and mean another. It knows you know better.
It is the greed inside your prayer.

In Keyholes

There is an apothecary of neighbors,
who live next door with a fury
of tinctures and wisecracks.
Everybody wants *a turn, a chance*
to throw insults like stones into
the pool. Talk behind our backs,
Can do that blindfolded, one arm
tied behind. The shovel-ready sunlight
is falling all over window sills, dusty
underneath, piled with last year's
holiday cards, never mailed.
It curves on the furniture, conversations
peeling-off in layers. Pearls and high-heels
weigh more than their ideals—
In backyards, there are noises,
jump-rope and dryers will make it
soft and nice. Rumpled little girls
getting cornered—The homework got left
in a puddle by the bad boy (now older,
now drunk!). Blackbirds on telephone wires.
New nieces and nephews, protecting
the secrets of infirm marriages, money woes,
broken kitchen tables, what gets said
that can't be put back in the bottle.
In the very end, our bodies become a whispering
of doctor's instruments—Privacy is the fever
that will loom at half-mast, tomorrow.
All the houses congregating to open up
a gateway to our anguish—Earmarked for
the landfill of last week's trash.
Our interiors deposited and undisclosed.
With our backs turned—This flashy society
of genes and germs, will relish to expose.

Family Therapy (I)

Mother/hood, a bald egg
in a grocery bag. The chromosomes
have their say, their stay in it.
The TV shows were all smiles
and cocoa. Environment.
Crisis management. My siblings
also hatched, perfect and imperfect.
The fitted sheets still warm
from the dryer.

I am my sister. I am my brother.
I am my brother's sister,
I am my mother's keeper.
I hold the secrets. I am the writer.
I am the sister of a schizo-
phrenic. My elder split—
My sister taught me how
to shave my legs, little slits of blood
left like a lunchbox in the mud.

I'm learning how to be a member
of my family, of my society.
I'm wanting a text book
on the matter. At the dinner table,
tension played *mirror, mirror.*
We all had our place
at the table. That space we wanted
to be erased from. Night by night,
it took us one course at a time.

I'm looking for a cure, because anguish
is harmful to live with. And yes,
I am a little pregnant. Set another
place? Erase another place?
I am my child's child, doomed
for failure. The father is my lover,
the sheets spilled his seed,
something took hold. When I opened
my eyes, my father held out a puppy.

Holes

White space as in flour
                        sifting

to my notebook, where the moth

I drew an hour ago, just flew off

                        the page.

It left a cone or a sphere—The space

around the margin, like the body's imprint

                        left on the bed.

The place I'm digging?— Unreachable,

                        or off-limits

as in a picket-line, or a picket fence.

For a moment, I want to see the in between,

                        awkward space

of a 3-legged dog. As a girl, I punched them

in jar-lids, to watch the metallic souls

                        of insects repeat,

repeat as a neon sign. At the last,

when the bathtub drains, do I remain?

The basin will dream itself

into something guttural, like my father snoring

in heaven—or taking up the bag-pipes,

                    instrument of death's

inflections. But he never said or told me:

Every how many miles do I rotate

    The tires?

The coat I wore to the hole

in the ground has gone to the moths.

                    So be it.

My insides lined with terrorists, this womb

a terrible coffin—Unborn. Undone.

                    Cigarettes burning

an armchair or an arm...The hole that the moth left

was an omission, rather an admission—

                    A portal or port-hole,

I let the insects fly out of the jar.

Zig-Zag

Don't worry, you'll know me
I'll be the one crouched beside myself—
Jewish Yankee in a Southern town.
I'll be the one saving for the next life—
    My folded grocery bags
    could extend for miles.
Bear with me, I'm saying this
for the last time—
I had been service oriented.
    I was the subject
of an experiment in derision—
    The sum total, splitting apart,
unrecognizable as a flea. I put out
    an all-points bulletin,
but still couldn't find myself.
    I can't draw a straight line
for the life of me. But really, I don't want
your sympathy. I'll wait my turn. I know how
    to suffer, that part is easy—
I'll be the one with my hands
to my ears—right before a china cup
    hits the tile floor. My head gathered
as a small, angry crowd. By and by, my sister loosed
her sanity like a glove. I've faked and faked it well.
    I hear our ancestors yelling
from the mental ward of hell. We are right to be afraid.
It's the job we're here to do. I'll be the one
    with my hands up in the air—
But then, how will I know you?

Rumors Fly

When the starting gun fires,
blowing out all the dull parts—
                Presume shotgun weddings,
Tin-cans clanking under dented fenders,
rusted mufflers, passing empty store-fronts,
                factories spooked with half-truths—
Until the hearse drops the homeless brides
at the next dusty bus-stop. *(bad manners!)*
On the 44th floor, other end of town,
                many mouths circulate
the dirt at the water-cooler
of desire. Rampageous offspring—kids made
                of secrets and incest, witness
when germs are slurred and shared as fact
on polished gymnasium floors.
                The whispers follow
arm-in-arm, teeth powdery white as cocaine.
When rumors fly, take only what is necessary.
Open windows, plash the spirit
                in red pomp,
like a new dress made from old drapes.
Hounds of gossip will clamor
to the surest thing—a burning barn,
                the *swastika* on your arm.
We'll store a primrose of boughs, passed down
from the numbered sandwiches
of our ancestors. *When rumors fly, someone*
                will jumble the digits into vowels—
stain becomes stone, live into love,
groves will roll into graves,
where names lie
                breathless under snow.

Vessels

What I know hangs in doorways
Beneath my eyelids,
    in the trick room
behind the turning wall—
    out of reach
out of earshot, out of date—
    the groan between desire
and restraint. Unlucky, I learned
    the hard way, what can be held
can be broken. We were knee deep
    in our pleasures—
when the hourglass spent
    its sure-bet of time.
I thought I knew the mirror
    but I was wrong—it knows
me better—my beginnings all resemble
    endings. Menacing, what I knew
poured over syllables like hot coals.
    I learned the phrases
as a call to my arms—

But I've had to learn that arms
    are used for both love and weapons.
When everyone else sang,
    I mouthed the words.
I knew the before, but this is the after.
    I know cut flowers will need
a vase of water—How am I to imagine
    that someday, after me, my son will die?
What I know I learned from a Grecian Urn:
    The myths of men will play out
in stone. I know trees are meant
    to hold the rain. Afterwards,
I'll learn about a throng of thousands
    crossing Whitman's Brooklyn Bridge—
holding tight their ruin of shoes.
    All I learned and forgot, tallied
and catalogued in the room beyond
    the room of knowledge.

What the Blind See

This afternoon my son came inside
with lost mittens, but two new friends,
Jack and Ellie. He said he met them
on the backyard swings—introduced us
the way the blind pronounce faces
with their hands. He serves them
strawberry soup & pickled pudding
with a pinky, held up. I listen to him think
out loud, *"Ellie likes pretty shoes,*
but Jack loves pennies 'n choo-choos."
He wipes his nose, looks them square
in the eyes and chooses to love
all of the above: *"Ellie's cheeks are round*
as a peach. Jack's knees are dirty
as plums." Like anything worth having,
I'll teach him chores, but not the snarl
of metaphors. He's learning to see
by degrees, category, departure of lines—
Girls are soft, then fold themselves
like fans. Boys hide frogs, then spread out
like a warm breakfast. In his cramped kitchen,
he's cookin' with gas. The wide night turns on
its darkness. Two empty swings, ample in the wind.

25

Picture This

Three sisters just from swimming,
bathing caps, fresh cut bangs—
sitting at the pool's edge. This safe notch
in time hailed like a taxicab in the rain,
and memory makes it sedate
as a lawn chair, quelled
                    and awash in *Technicolor.*
Think picket fences. Think polka-dot sundresses.
Smiles and lemonade implied
for later the same day. Imagine the mother
in tortoise-shell glasses. She never gets wet
above the waist, keeps her petite figure
                    like a secret thing at the back
of the drawer—for future reference.
Imagine the lens, one pupil behind
the lens. At home, two muddy shoes
depressed or manic at the back door?
Life offers possibilities—a kiss with
a fist or a salesman's pitch? Now tinctured,
                    with time, bereft of manners.
Viewer, if we knew then what
we know now, would we have kept a safe
distance, null time and space?
Would we have considered the mood,
lighting, TV channels, sofa positions?
                    The automatic pairing
of depth and perception.
The shadows are able to steal
a moment and lie, easy to snap
as *Tupperware. Viewer,* as long as
you're here, recall the ride home,
hot vinyl sticking to thighs, a fly buzzing
                    around the silence
between the noise, like a snag
in the upholstery.
Later the same day,
in matching sundresses, imagine
these sisters winching the knots
into tightly woven nests of macramé.

Google Me

Apparently, you've been going neck
and neck with all the enemy combatants.
It seems this rig you've lived in
and called your name has gone to

the smokestacks of insignificance.
By all accounts, You're living in the shadows
of a throng of selves—You're also an atheistic
pastor, dusting the pews with high-to-heaven

shoes. You're a sycophant gymnast, splaying
apoplectic contortions on the mat.
But in a nano-second, you're a biologist
pharmaseuticologist, *wanna-be* neurologist

looking for the sure demulcent cure.
You're a bald hair-dresser, who can't dye
her own hair. This must be what they meant
by a past life—You used to be a diet-diva,

but now you're a metro-sexual lawyer.
Who knew you'd be a 16 yr. old virgin,
growing expert in solitude and pain?
One day, you'll be a dead Gothic princess,

waiting for a graveyard kiss. You've been reincarnate,
fated to search your own tombstone. The ship
has gone belly-up—you're bolting the doors
to cordon-off a bottleneck of forsaken names.

We all have our standards. Haven't you earned
the right to the skin of your own name?—
Once upon a time, you were just a girl
running through a backyard sprinkler.

Crickets

Risking everything, they awaken you
to the night's unfinished business—Ear-worming
the dew with a quiet fury. Weary hitch-hikers snubbing
a ride to your *hit-and-run* childhood.
                         We were shirtless
and naughty in the back of his *Mustang—Jailbait*
 is a word in a song that will haunt you
at lunch-time. A thrum in your throat, a static radio of love
gone wrong.
                         The natal waiting room
was a loud jiggling of keys—then silent
as a kibbutz of prayers.
                         All the necessary evils were there.
A cough in another room, a nascent noise lifting
the fog like scraped paint from a door.
                         Your empty bed gone dark
and cold, a winter potluck. The trees make no apology.
Only the sympathy of wind-chimes, a child crying
on a swing. That dog you want to hold is hiding
                         in the cushions of memory—
Restless dog, still not housebroken.
(Someone impaling the upholstery.)
                         Wave it now as your passport
to the old country—(the way home by heart,
the broken bracelet left on the dresser
of your girlhood)—Loss and ache like the rain
falling from a pen and ink drawing you found,
someone else had crinkled
                         into sound and tossed away.

Birth Right

Born to know that feathers
on a bird's wing are wired for flying—
That the butterfly has lived
a previous life—Grass to leaf to sky—
Born to know to look for
higher ground—That the moon comes
in many variations, and at no admission price.
Born to know I have bloomed
from a bloodline. I could pick my lamp-lit aunt
out in a lineup—I know my own voice
in a crowd—and when I blow, it will whistle.
Born to know that a trout
can't mate with a rabbit, as Tevia said,
"Where would they live?"
My young son was born to know
all the songs to, "*Fiddler On The Roof.*"
I wonder what Einstein brought for show and tell?
Born to know that some things
call for ceremony, and some a puddle
of grief. The skin is a faithful guardian
if only for a short time.
Born to know that we'll never settle
our accounts—That the seasons are a paradigm
sometimes drenched in rain.
Born to know which *Monopoly*
token to pick on a snowy day—(Iron or shoe?)
That bus stations smell bad—And the poor are damned
to be the sweepers of the floor.
Born to know a slammed door
means someone is leaving—the last one out is jinxed.
Born to marvel at the ants
trudging over the anthill—That the landscape is crawling
with green places we've never been.

Born to sow these blessings
in wonder—because our longing
will never be quenched.

Part II

Family love is messy, clinging, and of an annoying and repetitive pattern, like bad wallpaper.
—Friedrich Nietzsche

Family Therapy (II)

We ignore the kinship of strangers
because we are seamed and stitched
together—our canopy for the long haul.
       This pathos has static and is stuck
like the plastic covers in the photo albums.
We are composed of posed facts
and time eludes us with
              Country Club smiles.
I wore patent leather shoes and polka-dot
socks from the bargain basement
of the *Family unmentionables.*
       In collusion, the hand-me-downs
have given birth to aunts, uncles,
and the rowdy cousins. My Family
needs an accountant for the bank
of DNA—which stands for,
       Do Not Abandon
Ship. We come from a long line
of liars and fools running off
with the silver — Because we are
Family, our inkless shadows
       have left no prints.
Let's recast the time when Aunt June
knocked on the back door, unannounced—
a wilted flower in her wilted couture.
       No worse for wear, all the way
from Miami, she came to bellow and shriek
like a freak teapot. Theory: Aunt June clocked
a few degrees south of center—
reviving our ancient fear that all roads
       lead to Florida.
This elevator is already full, thank you,
so I keep looking for a balcony
from which to drop. *The Family*
       is worried to death
that there are no happy endings.
But when push comes to shove,
our shadows will always make room
       for the next of kin.

Foundry

At the factory of lullabies,
fonts and DNA, a birthday book
was forged—fairy dust and pulp—
cherry perfume, loitering in spines
after curfew. We wave to ourselves
as reflections in a store window—
into a time that has already happened.
Deep forts erected from sheets,
blankets, terry cloth towels held by
nightstands and flowered beds.
When you laid out the Tarot
cards next to the pink-haired trolls,
I wondered if we were beings made
from other materials?—Caterpillar silk
of doll hair, crisp paper archived
from a tree. This is nature's perfection
hand-hewn with all the provisions—
Just a few flaws, throw the disease
into a jar. When they met by committee,
you were called to bigger things—
bell bottoms, peace signs, parties ending
in disheveled graveyards. Thin as
a paper-clip, your smudged lipstick
was cast with loneliness and lorn.
One night, the wind bit as strong
as a wolf with a paw in the threshold
of your dental records—A swath
of dress slipped out from the car door.
Two sisters, owls at the cotillion
of seeds and flowers. The cousins shiver
under the elm, our polyester nightgowns
buoyed up in flames—warehoused
forever by buttons and souls.

Letter to Metaphor

Soundless as a disc on a dot of snow
—Emily Dickinson

It goes without saying, there's something
for everyone. Remember the slut
of the multi-purpose room,
           legs spread and bearing
the burden for everyone—?
           Lipstick put on
for all the wrong reasons,
and all dolled-up for what
the bed of roses stole.
           A note was penned
by simile's hand—your first cousin
allergic at the ersatz country house,
flirting with images and glyphs.
           Ask for subtlety, you'll get
a mixed strip-tease every time.
No consequence, no punishment,
like when you helped write
           cheat notes on the inside
of my hand—the same naked hand
that braided hair, slipped off a coat—
traded in sex for a prayer.

Vacation

Suitcases packed, the dog carted off —We piled in the
paneled *Station Wagon* holding tight to our dream pillows.
A week-long life-style. The open road stretched out,
warm as comfort food. Rid us our ruts, our tangled roots—
A whole system concocted for consoling our wounds. No
seat-belts, giddy with candy wrappers, car games. Then
wishes were hushed on stars. Miles of roads, gas stations,
Vacancy signs—all pin-pointing the emptiness we left at
home. It's hot. The singing has stopped. The *Wonder*
bread sandwiches sweat in the Frigidaire cooler.
Tomorrow, my sisters and I will rummage seashells to find
the hidden secrets inside something so small.
O Technicolor, O Camera, please give us back our posed
snapshots of happiness and calm. We came to this
inosculate horizon to find smiles frozen in time—water
lapping at our ankles, like the dogs we left behind.

On the way home, a girl in pig-tails shows her tan line on a
billboard. (It's 1968, no seat-belts, no pedophiles?). The
smudge of soot on her buff cheek, like a scorch left
on an ironed shirt. Tonight at the *Holiday Inn,* we will be
doodling on the bed when the flickering black and white
TV wallows in muted grains of eidos: *"Martin Luther King*
was shot on a balcony at 6:01 p.m. at the Lorraine Motel in
Memphis." We will pack our souvenirs of grief for a sound
older than dinner—At home, the dog bellows a bluesy howl,
ache springing forth like cotton balls from the bottle.

You Know You're Alone

When the lips of snapdragons
play an anthem as the door
swings back open when
                your lover has gone.
You know it when assembling
your sins in a row and ticking off
your best and worst ones.
And you know when the small feet
                of silence conspire
in your ear—buzzing throng of insects
teasing your name. Sullen heart crumbling
like burnt cake no one wants to eat.
You know when the gibbous moon rises
                like an old rubbed coin—
and the band plays on without you. Imperceptible
vibrations of a distant telephone,
perched like a bird who
                forgot how to sing.
You only hear a somber newscaster
in a distant room—God has stuffed swaths
of cotton in tired ears. Is that why you've been kind
to your inner voices? You know it when
                you're hungry and lost
on a dusty road, but don't stop to look
for lodging—You've stopped waiting
to lay down with desire—At the wide gap
                where the future ends.
One rainy morning, all the guests left
without warning. You looked out the window
to where the water meets the door, and opened it
to a place of astonishment.

The Ties That Bind

Every day we destroy a little more—
          The news-crawl across a TV
of continents and foreheads—Throngs of stitched veils
let in an origami of light,
          like geishas unencumbered
by wrapped feet, or a profusion
of butterflies yawning in a meadow.
          Blame it on the idle
tongue factory of—I talked myself into this.
          Blame it on what corrupts us—
Slave-traders—pleasure seekers,
one and all. Roll out the red carpet
          for the moral code.
That pedophile mouse looked
          deader than a doornail
when they pulled back the cotton sheet
          from the whiskered corpse—
Instantly, the floor disappeared
          beneath us.

At the tipping point, breathe deep,
listen to the argument
          of the human drone
like a warehouse of foghorns
or a chorus of seamstresses
          lined-up in a row.
Our snagged fabric threads us
and then lets go—seamless
          as a shadow government.
The tortured ones will eventually pop
the cork out of the bottle—
In a kitchen, a quarrel ends with
a slammed door, then a face weeping
          in a bombed out window—
twice removed, across the 6 o'clock news.

Shelf-Life

I followed the invisible keeper
of the shelf—Languishing, dated
as dried inkwells in the lofty residuals
of antique malls. The past was a skin,
a trinket lined in satin, like an old school
Valentine someone finds in a drawer.
　　　　All the morticians
have thumbed their noses
at mortality—then pinched us into
distinction. *"No pearls before
swine, and Madam, please move
to the back of the line."* My pages
were immured like sacred parchment
in exotic rainforests—The sloppy words
went damp as motel towels, scrimmed
under a door.
　　　　One time I slammed that door
on my finger and sent the bats flapping
to higher ground—All my former thoughts
resembled smudged chalk or dead insects.
　　　　No harm done. I was the first
of my kind. These are the thousand reasons
we are inconvenienced on a dark planet
　　　　to be exiled from home—then stranded
at the corner payphone of the last century.
When I slipped on the ice at the rink
of the page, it was a sucker's sacrifice.
So tooth and jowl, you ask,
Now what? What now?

Dear Reader,

"...the youthful bloom of new books, which lasts until the dust jacket begins to yellow, until a veil of smog settles on the top edge, until the binding becomes dog-eared, in the rapid autumn of libraries."
—Italo Calvino

Do you recall when the pencil made us
fathom the unsayable? Foot-loose tools
of language—consonants and vowels
took their own sweet residual time.
Recall the hands,
how they played a part, almost
ancestral, fingers taut and hugging
the surface as if to a cliff. The tip
of pen, it too, touched a nerve—
Hand-stitched, an idea fixated
to a word, not like ornament,
but more like a risk—
a tight-rope walker's held breath.
It hushed and consoled us into
our aloneness—Led us through
the crawl-space of the family blood-line,
inchoate cave, hand-bag of self.
Oh Reader! Oh Writer!
The paper was loose-leaf, a dense forest
of suggestions. A medicinal arsenal,
as though someone turned out
the light, left a stain of tea.
Yes, a little scrappy,
oh ok, a rinky-dink circus if you must—
but it was the "I" skating, doing
loop-de-loops,
cordial as a doctor making rounds.
A spirit out of nowhere, a stroke
of good health—a little weary and love-lorn,
(holy sheet hides an ornery ghost)
no need for introductions,
intrinsic mind in hand—bridging the gap.

Table

For once, tell us your troubles—
turn your wobbly legs upside down
like an animal at rest. Your frank surface,
weary of being both the anchor
or the wedge—Where love and hate
sit across from one another, unchallenged.
Make no mistake, this is where
the education happens. Even the straw
lips of brooms hug close, waiting
for scraps, fighting the dog for
our tender sorrows. (Flotsam can be grim.)
Salving wounds—blueprints made,
mugs clinked at a good deed. Pencils sharpened
for the party invites, or a calculation
or a sliver of a thought. Wishes blown
into bottles hold a sound like tip-toeing
in the graveyard. Here we polish our
nails, to coyly hike hems for a date
that will get broken, or worse, forgotten.
Bones picked clean. We come to cut our teeth
on your pocketful of rings. All the dinner plates
rattle, testing their cracks with pathos
and glue. Listen to the echoed
noises of your life—Sturdy to hold a glass
half full of milk, our little miseries
newspaper worthy and too complex.
We are rapt like a quilt at your
secure location. Come now, pull up
a chair, be unburdened, rest here.

As Seen From Above

(for P.W., August 11, 2006)

While your mind is singing
the only song you know,
I'm folding the sun into drapes,
the drapes foreclose
on the lawn. You make a tent
        of your hands,
protect me from the elements.
In your palm, something along
the lines of a future tense.
I was the girl in a paragraph
of a simpler time—where words
were considered monuments.
Your face is lined
        as a roadmap, but your fingers
tell a different story. When I can't think
sitting down, you whistle to lighten
the load—a bird's song emerging
        after heavy rain.
All our belongings like luggage
thrown off a ship. The pillars of shadow
are tender on thighs and elbows.
Our mouths are housed
under one roof. We're wayward
pilgrims looking for the one window
light that calls us home.

Nest

Because there is a phone booth
where I want to be kissed swift
as a stolen car going nautical
in the rain—I was jinxed, put on love's
blacklist, flunked all the tests.
Got sent to the principal's desk,
(greasy comb and metronome)
for dreaming improbable dreams.
Kept a diary in my head about
the complexity of living rooms.
Doors creaked like sugar
to a toothache. Loneliness bodes tight
with a body stowed in a trunk.
But in this life there is still room
for heft and kindness—We found love's
office in a movie theatre.
I wept over a fish that reminded
me of my father. A bounty of sound
wooed us, all by a man sweeping
the silence, then moving it. Your fingers
wove something resolute into mine,
as if to catch a baseball or a snowflake
on the tongue. You would find my
best kept secrets. Crooked into
the top shelf of memory's
tree house, I found the letter
you carried with everything
gathered from the earth—string,
three theories of an argument, a lock
of hair. At home, there will be words
scratched in the walls of a shanty
lit-up beside a river—a kind of grace
nestled in, to protect us from
the elements and the answers.

God as a Character in the Room

Owning the world order—
The solo held post—Final night watchman,
almost Hitchcockian—
Ghost or guru,
                    All-knowing
in rooms where everything goes still—
But the lady at the window
is a hummer, in other words, she always hums—
no songs, just notes, humming
                    to give the silence
a voice. The moon or a blinking eye
follows us home—Did we see what we saw,
or what we were already looking for?
(Be careful what we wish for—)
                    In the omniscient glass
of hours, at the diner of time
where everything is dated,
                    nothing is sacred.—
Elvis and Jesus are one and the same.
It's ok, we're pagans, waiting for an excuse
to clank our cups—until we are served
Adam and Eve on a log—
                    Outside, on the busy street
a troubled noir of clouds—
where a brown-suited man
gets holed, not holy in a drive-by shooting.
                    Humming the news
at the kitchen sink, Eve had an alibi—
The moon or an owl perching
on a branch of snow,
                    saw everything perfectly.

Part III

What a distressing contrast there is between the radiant intelligence of the child and the feeble mentality of the average adult.

—Sigmund Freud

Family Therapy (III)

In this house of Ruth
clearness of mind is just
wishful thinking—
an unmade bed takes up
all the air in a room.
This illness was built
brick by brick,
but none of us knows how
to blow it down.
Our shame is seasoned
and matter-of-fact. We wear
bright clothes to trick the eye
into believing there is a reason
to dress in the morning—
We should have known
that something was seriously
wrong when the clouds
were calling us by name—
We hear the long squeal
of a train, before it finally
comes to a stop. Even the wolf
is sobbing. Our moods swing
easy as a top popped off
a soda can. We arouse
more than a little electricity
in a room. The family dog
can't fathom these domestic
complications. He eats and sleeps,
avoids eye contact, and hides under
the bed during storms.

Without a Visible Sign

(after music by Jan Garbarek)

Seed me the need to pair down, threaten
       six birds with one
stone. Indecipherable lists, breeding
       more lists—Remember when
the chalkboard scratched its weary head
in delirium, desperate for the proof,
       an empirical evidence
that *we were here!* Translucent shoal
of fish swimming a blue streak
       in the river that holds
my religion—and my house beside it,
the domestic institution
       of the soul.
The river is my lung, or the long green
dress I never got to wear to the prom.
       The crisp gown, still tagged
and left on the bed by my mother's guilt
like hush money clad in chiffon.
       Is there ever simplicity?
The wrinkled symphony—the river's violin,
the bullfrog floating with eyes closed
       like padlocks and waiting to awaken
to the night's uncertainty. The riderless
canoe spreads the inchoate word
       of mankind. My foot soldier
(prom-date) weary and hocking for war or fertility—
it's always one or the other. *Don't ask, don't tell.*
       Water and oil will be the elements
that make us kill. I'll spend the rest of my days
telling my story, someone else will tell theirs.
       The prints will be left—
You have to forget everything
You know to write poetry.

TV

When you awoke / the war was on—/Fuzz and static / B.52's
of quiet / not like *Shhh, the baby is sleeping/*
but the manic dust / post shoot-out—/Cowboys blowing on
guns / or condoms at 3 a.m. / blue rill of night— / It looks
back / at you / steely eyes / ears plugged / smug like a shark,
gnashing. / We are told to suck / on all its nipples / Dinner
served /on a silver tray /on parent/teacher night / It squawks /
rattling every gold /filling in the neighborhood/ Antennaes
swaying like the tongues /in electric thunderstorms/ /Little
box of tinkers / with so many voices / talking all at once/ O
rubber doormat / it seduces stupidity/ has little sympathy /
prattling mandates / soliciting / telling us to see / many sexy
theatres / in our small eyes / *Eat a pretzel / pop a can/ take
some Prozac / Be rid of acne!/* and every human / quirk /
imagined / It tells you to laugh and screw on track /
Broadcasts / the hidden / motif of wants—/ Commands us /
to flip through / every channel / to surgically remove / every
crafted / origami heart—/ This gangly box / intoxicating / the
shame and shock / imbibing on / the envoy of our pain /

Vacuum

Wound tight, I'm not in the mood
for rumor, just a brief reprieve
from a life consumed—
Gearing up for the purge and suck,

the hot air censoring what is
useless and paper thin.
The lint in my voice keeps me

from saying, "Get a life, get a life,"
and that bears repeating when
the voluminous Tulips are in full bloom.
I've put all else on the waiting list.

If my body had a noise to see
itself through, would this be
the cacophony? A sweeping prestige

like the director's camera zooming in
to the art of the weave—soiled rug
that is thankless as a spoiled husband
and demands my undivided attention.

Under the bed ruffle and through
the brush, where my hair has depilated
into a rat's nest. For a brief season

of illusion, I can pluck out the husk
of my sadness. Because life aims to sting
not like a bee, but more like a boxcar passing
through a womb—like the laborious mothers

who give over their lives. My ancestors
beat out their rugs with the silence
of brooms. We all need something to blame.
Looking for absolution in the dust, but the mess
of life escapes my wrath—as in a memory I have

of a couple who embraced so long on the sidewalk,
their bodies could only be a receptacle for grief.

Voices

Then we turned and parted company,
my voice and me—It was played back
by the machine, to introduce itself to itself.

Each larynx like a snowflake, no two the same.
Collectively, the voice is the kitchen table
of home. If it could, it would jump out

and bite you on the mouth. Conflagration
of shame, so hot and high-pitched it will shatter
a teacup in your hand. If only God would clear

his throat to be a troubadour to the moon?
Oh tenor of our connection, the little
blessed box to the soul. *"So late, so late,"*

the voice cursed knocking at the door,
*"I should have phoned, should have phoned.
Damn to the dial-tone and the vacant howling wind."*

A déjà vu of sound serves as translator
for the insane—when too many sit
on the head of a pin? Short-wave to the past ones

that haunt me—Loud and clear, the principal intoned
over the intercom, as we recited *The Pledge
of Intolerance.* Our voices rising like a football field

of cloud formations. All together, the boos and cheers
could be a lethal weapon. In bed later, at the porch
of my ear, so cordial, *"Good night, good night,"*

and lets the breath escort it out the door.

Bernadette in Arches

(after a photograph by Jim Stroup)

*"A photograph is a secret about a secret,
the more it tells you, the less you know"*
—Diane Arbus

Here the columns imply action
deprived of action,
like a letter that never arrived.
The postscript would have
implied a different circumstance.
Inside pillars, she is the rind
of religion. Circles and arcs
are not forsaken, but a nosegay
for the host of spirits in her mind.
Her tablecloth has labored
over generations of banquets
and secrets spoken to no one,
but louder than words
could ever say. Marble implies
structure...implies force...
implies an echo of a voice
that called her late for dinner.
Once, a voice sang in a forest
and someone cut down a tree
for the very first time. Someone else
arranged the branches into architecture—
Into where *man* implies *woman*....
implies *pitcher*....implies *shelter*....

Etude for the Asking

Don't fix what's already broken.
Museum of sound, my voice
caterwauling on the machine,
in an empty room.
Tsk, Tsk, too clairvoyant.
A vertigo of doors: *"I can't be reached,*
can't be reached." I am the ventriloquist's
worst nightmare, hoarse at the beck
and call of a plastic mouth.
Crying is a useless activity,
it makes my face ugly, stricken
as a wasteland. Why this salty laundering?
Swallowed nail holes, yesterday's puddle
all dried up. A lapsed negative furled
to a question mark. Museum of film,
the skin remembering itself
for the lake of celebrity. Shelved into
a brick wall, as all those abandoned
gas stations marooned by time.
Hence, Chaplin's dark brim spoofed
the silence, a swift cane, *Hitler mustache*
thrust like a flag. His treatise of slapstick,
heave-ho-tricks fooled our pain
only as long as the tail chased the dog.
Don't fix what's already forgotten.
Starved for attention, attrition,
museum of here and gone—
a licked envelope at the tail-end,
vaccine for the deceased,
trial and error, *Spaghetti Western*
winnowed to dust, a lost language re-furbished
by chatter, chinks of human teeth.

You Should Question:

When lipstick marks show up
on hankies that aren't your own.
When motel signs say, *"Pets Welcome."*
Question when dental hygienists
go poking around in the century
of your mouth, gold-diggers all,
for your crowned jewels of chloroform
and anguish. Question the fear
that makes you question—
     Where do we go from here?
Question elocutionists with speech impediments.
Reflect later, when the doctor says,
"This won't hurt a bit." Beg to pardon,
when the sofa insists *this* isn't *your* home.
When the glossy packaging promises
to pop out cellulite like bubble wrap
(until the fat seeps back like fog under a door)
     Scratch your head
at that fast talking hipster from the telethon
for the *Golfer's Relief Fund?* And tread lightly,
when the night wakes you to your
'inner child' and says, *"the case for 'privacy'*
is closed." It's okay to show true alarm
when Ayn Rand winks at you in a bikini
     from the grocery store check-out—
Promising ten ways to wax and attract
an alpha-architect. You'd better first vet
that existential treatise that proclaimed
God said: *"Go ahead, go ahead, go ahead*
and strike me dead!"
     When your paradigm works
backwards. When your sloshed friends sing
to you in party hats! When you don't like
what you see in the interior mirror.
When your happy pill begs for
a refill—Okay, then worry out loud when your heart
     goes cloudy and pencil still.

Terror in the Streets

The alienation of others
Wears on. Between us,
Generals count arrows in a quiver.
—Adam Zagajewski

This year *camouflage* is *in*.
Every gas mask hides a face.
Riots of antics, botched semantics.
Roots beat in the ground with tainted blood.
On cue, they died with their boots on.
Roll up the town at 5 p.m., roll up the shantytown.

Inside job—the interiors have no walls.
Not in this life, the flag said to the flower.

Ticks picked off scalps like fleas on elephants.
Hell on earth—the literal tropes the earth.
Each grave used to be a parking lot.

Salute the new crop of suicide-patriots.
The news has a title and a theme song.
Rain usually leads to rust or rumor.
Elbows exposed, the nuns show skin.
Enough blame to go around.
Tanks moving on a wing and a prayer.
Snow on steeple, phalanx of dead people.

Country Mouse, City Mouse

She said:

Dear Cousin, I wish you could see
This autumnal light—
Tugging—at the turnips—
Like a window curtain—
Tugging—Like an eye—
The seeds have eluded—
These alluvial streams—
Like a spell—The dust *poofed*
From an ancient letter—
Thus and so, flower
is to stem is to stamen—
Oh busy bee—Examining
The fruits—of your last requests?
(Oh for spacious skies—)
A thrush of pollen—
The clouds are pin-striped
and have made a pledge—
To love? —This letter is a field—
This field is an accordion—
Of green—*Same old, Same old—*
But glorious—just the same—
In the barn, nostrils are flaring—
Eyes blink—A contrail of steam—
A phone—rings?—Is it you
Between the crackle—and static? —
Are you man or mouse—?
Squeak up! Remember us
In the shadows—where time was
A rumor—barely mentioned—
Someone's crazy uncle—
TV zapped & pajamaed in the attic—
The birds were humming—
Leaves lit with denunciation—
Spiders spun the webs of our—
*Salutations—*Dear You,

Over the horizon—My moon—
My mouse, snoring—
Like a wolf—in sheep's clothing.

He said:

Cousin dear, I miss the language
Of our fire-escapes--Rickety—
Rickety—Because home—
Is the one place—
We've never been—
Text and Hypertext—
The thieves and sluts—
Have gone looting—
I was given my pink-slip
In the brown-out—An invite
To war—I miss the subways
Doing Loop-de-Loops—
Eyes—averting—Eyes—
Like an underground
Subtext—Mugger is to
Stranger—Is to held
At gunpoint—Is to pinned
To terror—While pigeons peck
Missives into brown paper bags.
The architecture—Is an archive—
Is an arbitrary record—?
If one blast—can change—
The cityscape? If I squint—I can imagine
Your fishnets—(Multiple choice—or,
fill-in-the-blank?) *Kiosk is to Kamikaze*—
Was to—I was just a white-collar guy—
Now I'm kicking up
Cowboy dust?—5,000 miles—
Oh Hyperbole—Oh Cousin,
I miss your pink slip—
And your frisky tail—
Remember the power outage—
And how we made moon-shine
in the apartment—where we mouse-sat?
Are all the chewed wires—
Star-crossed Lovers?—Last seen,

Their fedoras were tipped—
Across America—Lonely as
Phone booths—Receivers off, dangling—
Polished black and empty—
As a dead man's shoes—

Elegy for a Scarecrow

October's henchman has bled again.
Evenly the straw is strewn
without retribution or shame.

An amplitude of human contact
stitched into the farmer's flannel shirt,
that still smells of apple cores, smoke and hay.

This hired hand without pay, here to usher
in bounty and harvest, where yearning is heard
intermittent as an owl in the barn.

At first frost, face down, he knew his place
and his art, presiding over compost and rue—
the last of the soup stirred in

a lonely widow's kitchen. Last spring
the children and ghosts of her grown children
sprinkled the seeds in all the wrong places—

but a garden grew just the same.
A snow of willows. The landscape shivers.
He never said a word, but she looked for

his company, understanding his serious business
with the weather. Befriending pumpkins
in midnight sun. The crows are inconsolable,

their wings leave stains across the moon.

Part IV

What's love got to do with it?
                                         —Tina Turner

Family Therapy (IV)

It is the thing we always fail
to mention on all the forms—

the despotic voices dancing off
the charts, and on the trail

of our acrid ancestors, haphazard
and lorn, sniffing us out like cadaver dogs.

Our chromosomes flirting
on the cordless phone—Diseases of the heart

and kidney are just the body's bric-a-brac.
Incorporeal or obscene? We are the doctor's worst

unexplained nightmare. And we never speak
of the Endocrine glands—Unsavory

secretions passed down like the heirloom
nobody even wants. We are a Rogue nation.

No country or comfort zone. Inhospitable bedrooms,
where our parents detonated bombs, blamed

the groping in-laws. Our family trait is to remember
only the good times, like a last blown kiss

at the door—But more like a breath
blown over a bottle, forever haunting

the offspring. Hush, we'll never tell,
yet deep down we know, the mind's pain

is the last inconsolable and extra gene.
Rabid dog in the school yard—

Mean and mad and frothing.

In Plain Sight

*Incomprehensibility has an enormous
power over us in illness...*
—Virginia Woolf [On Being Ill]

I am certain of only one thing—
I am a team of (n)one.
      In the lineage, all things pass
through the kitchen, the mouth, origin
to the tribe. Smudged surfaces claim every trace
in the family cell—I moistened my toothbrush,
      it came back with germs of madness—
Verdant and wet, just this side of the doormat,
pale footsteps are left at the ajar
of an argument. One June afternoon,
a feud erupted (in the frozen food section).
It was hot as a dog's nap. Then, a baby cried out
      like a roadside bomb.
I kept smiling at the cashier, thumbing
bruise-less fruits, counting the dated
canned goods. It took hostages, sealed windows,
      taped my mouth
shut with sugar and pleasantries. I kid you not,
it pawned off my jewelry, blood diamonds
of /t/rust. I screamed out loud,
      but nobody heard.
I need to mind what matters most—
My sister needing a phone call,
my husband an apology, the time to watch
my son fumble a soccer ball down a muddy field.
      I am so clumsy
to the people I love. I've slid my tongue
on the sharp end of the conversation.
I am the form built to last, but made with
      cheap labor and parts.
(Do you *wanna trade your troubles for mine,*
yours are manageable, and state-of-the-art.)
The dog watches my son when I'm not home—
      (I mean, *home*, but not).

Order/Disorder/Order

By golly, you can go crazy anywhere
    and never know when your finger
will be caught in a door. No denying
    that pain. *Good cop? Bad cop?*
My thoughts were shipshape
    until they sank inside
the hole of a doughnut, later detained
by a traffic light. Their thoughts were flimsy
as a house of cards. Folly, riots in the streets,
'tis why churches were erected.
    Feng shui: the art of placing
pleasing arrangements, until they agree
    to disagree. *Disclose my unbearable
junkyard of mental debris?—No dice.*
The afternoon had a picnic.
The afternoon had a 10-car pile-up.
    Never a dull moment.
Tweedle-dum & Tweedle-dee,
    what began as a smile, defaulted
into a frown—Do the mouth's borders
    own our comfort zones?
Systems of justice, systems of punishment;
the first system was that of the parents,
replaced by the Dewey Decimal System.
    Everything is relevant.
    Everything is irrelevant.
Brick and mortar, a nervous disorder,
marriage, divorce, work to lay-offs...
    After the sundial, clocks were devised
for the mind's original origami—
    neatly folded creases *organized*
into a system of belief. Our public menace
is time's flustered dance,
        where nothing was left to chance.

A Sign of the Times

Gotham City gawks in awe
    at the new raw data, or history's short
retention span. All the white cartons
    of Chop Suey have been banned,
instead, *Kentucky Fried Children* were left
    for Sunday's supper. As civilians,
should we save the best or worst for last?
    It always comes down to a clash
of maps. *All bets are off.* This frenetic
    whirlwind looks to cook the books,
stir the soup frothy, until it's red, white,
and stew. *Validate my parking ticket,*
my compatriot. It's a rat-race out there.
    In here, a red/black interior
only *Francis Bacon* could understand.
    When all is said 'n done,
I am a gumshoe. No I am my website.
    No, I am Ashleigh Banfield
doing Nancy Drew, *doing* the news.
    Angora sweater, buxom boobs, librarian
    glasses to match Martha Stewart's *blues,*
(oops, I meant, hues). How we tweak and yearn
    for a lunchbox, or a lunch made
by *familiar hands.* Where was I when they replaced
    Walter Cronkite with Oprah, Inc.?
Then everything worthy became few
    and far between. They informed me
I needed a stamp for renewal, or was it approval—
    to visit the Tomb of the Unknown Soldier?
My bags checked at the body's station—
x-rayed to the nth. My razor and talcum risked
    death by lethal injection, or a fine-tooth comb.
The laser-gun did a *trompe l'Oeil,*
    but I couldn't blame this one
on my mother. Bulk-mail vanished
    into thin air, later captured by a ship
of pirates, or a virtual ship of fools,
waiting for their ship to come in.
    Eye-patched *palookas*
with whisky-breath looting the neon sea,

or *the devil taking his hindmost?*
We are castaways, getting lost to shrunken faces,
    further out on the barge of dark coats,
longing for something lamp-lit and constant,
    a pencil scratching its surface.
We are platonic, pell-mell, a statistic
    without a green card, or a greeting card
to tell us of *"The Shape of Things to Come."*
    I'll still take Ornette's copasetic riffs,
over Orlando's, *Tie a Yellow Ribbon,* any day.
    Let the music be arranged with no strings
attached. *You'll be told when it's over—*
Kaput, the fat lady sneezed thru the song,
    or the last loop of film.
All our red hearts beating unabashed,
    a twenty-one gun salute to the suicide
shoe-bomber, hung 'n drooling...
    And just as I suspected,
they told me to *let go of Elmo,*
    "Over my dead body, isn't the cold war
over (out-of-sight, out-of-mind, behind
    the ironic curtain)?" So I bought an over-
the-counter cure for the common cold,
    but just the same, caught *the virus*
going around, I think from a friend
    of a friend of a friend.

Unreliable Narrator

At the back of my throat, my impeccable
voice is a factory of cadences
and fabrications, when the will takes on
    a life of its own—
A canary's song, gone shrill
as a car alarm. These hounds
are bloodthirsty for a shadow to chase,
    never to catch up
with themselves. Let me spit a rue
of victuals into my shoe—
I'll tell the improbable mocking
tales that my mother warned against.
    The scarf trick of words
are only illusions saturated in
corn starch and fatty acids.
My wayward story shipped off
like sailors flexing their hulls—
and lose their erotic fables
to the teeth of the sea.
    The real truth was air-lifted
from the scene of the crime.
I'm just a landscape painter
with an ear for a garage-band:
"No, I've never colored my hair.
Yes, these are my real nails
and breasts."
    Do the math, I'm only 29.
What contract? I swear that kid
just fell from the top of the stairs.

    I swear, I didn't mean to share
your secret, it just slipped out
like a fever, like a lunch tray
from my hands."
    I'll tell you a lie
that will make you wince
and cry—My voice like a gas can,
sets the match to flame.

In A Parallel Universe

There are two little girls
in four pig-tails left at the pit-stop

of an abandoned gas-station,
waiting for the high school band

in Kansas or Kuwait—Our Kismet
is passing through a loud sound barrier,

nonchalant as a cereal box in
a church fire, or is it the coldest porridge

left by Goldilocks, on a table where pages
blew out the window, while a train passed through

the Encyclopedia Britannica, volumes A-Z.
Steam whistles, and a red velvet cab car reveals

the desires of a bank teller, or a bald widower,
pronouncing, "There's no draft to this war!" The band

can go back to football—which is how we pulled
elegy from the Eagle's beak, or was it effigy?

On the other side of the mirror, we will be stalked
by the lies we told. In a field of pumpkins and urns

a child is weeping with the cows, they stare at us
astute as busboys clearing plates and bowls. Our voices

went home without the key-note speaker, the clouds are
held up by toothpicks—A china shop, we don't dare enter.

Rooms

In my Father's House there are
many mansions.—[John 14:2]

These are the voluminous *Who's Who*
of unruly rooms, too full
of themselves. Notice the malcontents,
      nosing around for your undying attention.
Watch the ones that carry big sticks.
Avoid the eyesores not for the faint
of heart—Our cheap plates thrown
      like gloomy confetti. Keep at bay,
the hedonistic corporate rooms—
groomed into adulterous *sweetheart deals,*
where rooms are in bed
      with other rooms. That said, some rooms
are the picture of health. On a first-name basis,
and all about a feng-shui of breathing.
Once adorned, but now moth-eaten; remember
      when the tie-dyed curtains
had a vision and a moral compass?
The rooms where *I tell my people*
to call your people, but your people

Never call back! Stamped and approved,
distrust the rooms with *cherry-picked*
intelligence. The anterooms of anterooms.
      Ballrooms of children locked-up
in pageants of sad seductive
clothe styles. Stoic rooms that need
      a heart to heart—then corner us into
telling the truth! Mud-rooms where dogs lie waiting
for the key to turn. Bathrooms where someone
is coming of age—dangling a coat hanger.
      Rooms that are *dead-ringers*
for other rooms. Some talk their way out
of a jam.—The pleasure was all theirs!
Others are slated to be brainstorms,
      but have no threshold
and no door—A shrine of cobwebs,
a string of lanterns light the way
      to the last resolute room.

Face Book

It should come as no shock, our faces
as books, our faces the envy of
broken down clocks—Right-brain, left brain—
                    Let us be plugged in
at every turn, in every orifice.
This is our body! This is our office!
                    Staple every button-hole
that is latchkey and sad. Credentials culled,
there's no turning back now.
We're here to be cut and pasted.
Prepare us to be a billboard
                    blessed by the waste
of a flightless bird. The toasters are now
behest of prints left from a lover's
scorched breakfast. Too much work!
So stack our shelves with a library
                    of perfect smiles.
Salacious minds need routine, packaged
as shiny shrink-wrapped trinkets.
Screens screaming for sex kittens
and war porn—take the place
                    of breakfast and love.
Honk if you're lonely and your wardrobe
resembles a caption, wearing white
in winter—such poor taste!
                    Don't fret, an underling
took the place of your former self.
Pupils plaited and distal, the story
and the people got ransacked out—
exchanged for a remote page
                    of faceless doubt.

And So the Joke Goes

A man walked into a bar
                        To change the subject
on instinct or on a lark...
                        We wanted a change
of venue, leave revenue alone—we've had enough
                        of same, *same old.*
When the altercation occurred
                        we were caught unawares,
like *a pie in the face—Rolling up His sleeves,*
                        The jokes told and told
to the last one standing. The awful laugh of truth
                        spooked like the shock-awed
scene of an accident. Off-course, North to South
                        our naughty sailors crossed.
The koochy-koo of kraft walked into a mousetrap.
                        The subject was now the predicate—
As if putting on the wrong shoe.
                        "Can't have it both ways, dupid."
There's a sucker born every minute or cycle, what was it?
                        A serious matter, nevertheless.
Change is on the horizon—the sun is under occupation.
                        Bearded now, he told the one
about the Priest, the Buddhist & the Cleric,
                        who went to the *holy* circus
to see the dyslexic rabbi who said, "Yo," and proposed
                        to an Arabic acrobat with
a run in her stocking—Oy! Nothing sadder.
                        With a wink and a nod, we saw
the humor, but didn't get the joke—our solemn spectre
                        of fear changed everything—
A man walked in—Who had the last laugh now?

Frankenstein Meets Francis Bacon

It's only the little deaths to worry about,
when the guests' coats have left the empty bed.

When trees retreat to their forsaken contour—
Our thin skins lament the leaves

like a shaken loss of faith. And when lovers spat
without the slightest provocation,

holding tight to their walls of art—
recompense, as in a silent auction.

And yes, you should worry when your wallet
has fallen into the wrong hands

on a subway platform. Our handkerchiefs
awash in the bombed-out streets of civilization.

The monster that is made up of both
Mother Nature and God, has gone

completely haywire—And we're left to pick up
the pieces of mankind. Pray as we must

to dig through the little deaths,
which are the ones to grapple with.

In bed, the couple always turns to where
their paths will never cross—

Distant lamp on a bedside table
like a train pulling out of the station.

Afterwards, the snow falls futile and light
on the houses and hillsides—

to mute the fluent human pain
of when there's nothing left to say.

Pundits and Prophets

> *Ladybug, Ladybug, fly away home,*
> *Your house is on fire,*
> *and your children are gone—*
> —September 11, 2001

Dear God—
Business as usual,
but their daguerreotypes move
among us—lit inversions
like refrigerator lights refusing
to go out. Our requisite souls
going about our business
to less than what matters
to make matters worse,
this spasm of wreckage,
cordoned off—button, burnt shoe,
forensic toothbrush, birthday photo
(small boy in pointy hat).
Dear God—
How have we prepared
for this havoc? Were we those
children bringing the silver-wrapped
canned goods for the needy
at Thanksgiving break?—If only to
remember the pilgrims, carrying
their gear and personal effects
on boats not jets, until they landed
here, in *real time*, before the news
made non-sequitors of our artifacts.
Minute bits of print had a fanfare
in the funeral sky. Below, a phantom
hat-plume of smoke.
Dear God—
Give us the all clear. Give us
a structure that absorbs
its impact. Lamps. Pens. Notepads.
The desk has become a foxhole,
the last ash. Dear God,
In you we trust? A dillar, a dollar,
a 10 o'clock scholar. The pilgrims wash
their hands for good measure,
and someone goes on with his tennis game.

Caribbean Fishing
(after a photograph by Jim Stroup)

Six figures, six silhouettes
    in the ocean sunset—
A red so hot it will burn
bullets in your eyes.
These bare-chested men
are flexible and dark, they shimmer
    like the fish writhing
under a thunder-clapped sky.
On this island, *race is* present,
but unannounced
like a long shadow falling
    across an empty room.
In another context, these same men
might be mistaken for
a platoon of soldiers, feet blistered
    and far from home.
Brother to brother, counting
contours of bodies in the dusk.
    In another story,
on another shore, the women
are discreetly hanging laundry lines
    of yellow ribbons—
then cleaning the fish
and laying them out to dry.

Divided We Stand

Here we ruminate on divisions—Arrivals,
departures, the way relationships get cordoned

off—a property condemned— an argument, or a table
we have to walk around. Call it a framework,

a narrative that gets proofed into a pastoral storybook,
then collapses, mimsy as a paper-doll, or faith itself

minus the gods. Time pokes us, claims us, felt but unseen,
like an acupuncturist's needled touch. Divided by our

pockets—Ideals spilled at glittery parties, where pain
and guilt are lit up like after-dinner cigarettes.

Divided is not the same as *divorced* or *replaced*,
more like the linens dragged through the mud to shake out

the pixie-dust of life? Divvied up like the loud presence
of quiet, just before the shatter of applause.

The way architecture defines the space, a context revealed
in a pixel on a screen, which affords no margin

of error, none—Fragile is that balance, as if to remind us
we are here to open every door, turn handles, push borders

to unlock a kite-tail of grace—A staircase, a soap opera
of Gospel that never ends, appears like a prop to chronicle

the travesties of our lives. Aches that shield us, creased
and folded many times like old maps. Backyards divide us,

We are a nation of troubled hearts, leaning against
the electric fences of our soft animal arms.

Part V

"To put the world in order, we must first put the nation in order; to put the nation in order, we must put the family in order; to put the family in order, we must cultivate our personal life; and to cultivate our personal life, we must first set our hearts right."
—Confucius

Family Therapy (V)

Ok, so which came first, groceries,
or Genesis? The check-list is never
short-lived—This chaos was sturdy,
built to last. Seeds into seedlings—
The problems, no mincing words,
                    are twice engorged
at all elaborate family gatherings.
Funerals, mitzvahs, weddings—
we always get *The Group Rate.*

                    First-come, first-served—
boredom sets in, perches just a hair from
the lips of our daily details—(blemished
fruit baskets, fatwa of half-eaten cakes.)
The neighbors are minding their own business,
but they think we should 'mow the grass.'

                    You combed my hair, I dreamed
you were Elvis or Zeus or Moses?—Thrilling me
through rooms of exotic rugs, then rooms
of diapers and mops? *(Love is messy business!)*

                    Caught red-handed, we *played house*
poorly in an abandoned love shack, (sand in the all
the crevices of our pants), until *play* turned
into germs, a snotty toddler!

                    Close the door to desire?—
A voice thrummed in my ear.
Were we put here to hone, nest,
take-up permanent residence

                    to be the busy keeper
of appointments?—You combed
my hair, and words went silent
as potted plants.

                    I washed off my make-up.
Let memory's heroine cast a glance,
tell her own story about my navel,

                    fleshy teabag that reminds me
of the sadness that is language, the sadness
that keeps us human—keeps us from being
immune. Now I make lunch sandwiches
with lust in my heart and cellophane in my hands.

                    I am invisible, a *Plasma TV.*

79

My family of origin will always see me
an 8-year-old girl, no matter how old I become.
My husband and son see a woman scraping
gum from shoes, folding towels, salving wounds.
                    Only the dog sees the whole
picture, but he's too busy remembering yesterday's
garbage, the nuanced olfactory of a shoe
in the road, the tribe of his bone—a thousand years
buried by his ancestors.
My dog descended from wolves, the longest howl
I know next to train and fog horns.
                    I am invisible, but fully loved.
I rather like it, being an orphan.
I've learned to keep quiet—
to protect the self, the way my mother
slip-covered the sofas in 1968. I only write
                    when no one is home.
My son has never seen me *do it, write that is,*
as if *It* is a derelict act. I've kept these records
in a slip-cover of the page—a quiet song hummed
under the breath. A life lived in another life.
Virginia Wolf sifted rocks in her pockets
and went missing in the sea.
                    Let bygones be bygones.
Ok, so I laughed an a funeral once
when no one laughed back?— Papa Morrie
winked at me, fresh from the plot
of *the family business.* He was lit
and just about to tee-off, have the last
                    dead-pan laugh
and head to God's healing Spa in the clouds
of faith and contraband. God will fight
the good fight of dogma and politics
with Papa Morrie, (drinking whiskey, Turkish Coffee
from the old country, cracking nuts,
talking the talk about connecting
the dots— thru this gene pool
of miscreants, passage of rites, marriages
of inconvenience). But we'll always take
the good with the bad, to remain with *our own kind.*
                    Make no mistake,
when it thunders above, God (or is it the devil?)

tempts a naughty wife—Nana Ida turns out the light.
All the children safe asleep
　　　　　　　in their family of beds.

Exogamy

I always get it wrong, the timing—
like a focus group gone awry. No stopping
this manifest grind! Tonight, my corner
of the self needs tending, your undivided
attention—Fresh coffee resins at 2 a.m.!
O Busy hum of daily living—
Bills to pay, picture books
to put away. It's a full moon, the knights
are laying their swords down (after bath-time).
Dirty fingernails will be squeaked clean
as rubber ducks. Now, all my ghosts nudge me
to miss you—Though you're right here,
washing the cups, wiping down the canisters.
Going rogue, the chromosomes never
looked back—I remember that part of myself
falling into a cab, out of bad weather.
My apartment, the epitome of a car horn,
honking for no one. In this life,
there are train wrecks, bulging jungles,
dinosaurs parading on all the carpets.
Is the primitive kiss sent to our son in sleep,
the preface to a book, or the broken
chain-letter to history?—Whole kingdoms
stationed to collapse. My body
looks for refuge. Long barge at the entrepot
of desire—Then you'll arrive with
all the right supplies. For an hour,
the dragons will threaten only
the rooms where our loved ones
have just left—Their pains hidden
deep as a soldier's invisible wounds.

When Homer Roams

It's pointless calling, my thin voice
caught like gossip gone missing
from the laundry-line of home.
           I'm in no position
to give advice—You have all the knowing
ahead of me. Ears tipped into a tarot card
of portents—Oracle of scent and ethos—
drawn to the outskirts of puddle, leaf,
carcass, anything decayed, snowflake.
           This is your work,
it's serious business! With every breath,
willing to face death. You hear the sounds,
the vibrations once removed
from where I am not—like just missing
the bus from the bus stop.
           You'll wait for the kill,
steady, patient as a slow
drip in the well. That carefully made
lining and rill of your jowl flutters
with the nuance of butterfly wings.
The extra flap of skin always expecting
           company—the way we keep
a roll-out sofa for guests. Excuse us our
patio furniture, safe anchors, the area rugs
where you've kept vigil hold the habits
of our remorse. We know how to hold
a camera, we know how to visit
the sick with soup and gifts.
           We're only human.
Dog of the hearth. Wolf of the wild.
That long yowl is an anthem
unto itself. Stretched out, a rambling train
after the rains. Short days to night.
           My voice calling, beyond the doormat,
the smoke-plumed town, where the lights
are shutting down, and your prints
pander to us—we have no clue.

Phantom warrior showing us
how to bring the words
            back to their bones.

Diminution

It isn't easy being me,
breathless and hell bent
on rhapsody—My heartfelt sorrow
on the radio is backlit and infectious,
the way music makes our heads turn
to find our partners—Otherwise,
we dance alone. It's just as well.
My voices often speak
at the same time. Needless to say,
      This has consequence.
I'm an old-fashioned
hard candy, I don't dissolve
evenly—How large my want is,
how small. I talked myself into this.
I'm just an inch shy
of imploding—Ten thousand
pieces sprouting the self's
confetti across the wide sky.
I was a necessary justification,
but slim as a bar-code.
      I am a mass disappearance.
From the earth, I'm blinking
at the insects scrawled legibly
across the lawn. I'm a morsel
here to become something more
than I am. I'm the lozenge, buttering
up the tongue—sharp as a cat's claw.
The quick hand of childhood
      saw me to the door.
So pardon me if I forgot
why I came. A slow pen
in the palm of my hand.
Let me bend your inner
ear, because even this paper
needs body-weight—heft, the dent,
the fleck of having been there—
if only, in the smallest sense.

Hillsides

(after Philip Guston, *Untitled*, ink and acrylic, 1980)

The store clerk was gone in ten seconds
after the 30 rounds—blood spattered on
the welcome mat, soda coolers, cash register.
From the manhole in the studio, *Brian Williams'* voice
seeds my living room (*Brian*, who I know so well
but have never met). The blood so thick
in that storefront it makes me think
about brushstrokes piled in a heap
draped sly as Klansmen—Then I see
detainees at Abu Grahib, fowled
in brown paper bags. The silver screws
and gawky nails that turn to fists,
if you stare long enough
at the painting—Guston's cartoon
versions, haunting all our worst fears.
Every night, *The News* stock-piles
in my living room. The pink rubble
and gray maw of Japan floating off
falling rocks, buildings dislimned.
White clouds that aren't clouds at all.
Dust flaring off the *TV* from muddied
combat boots, that have brazed and combed
hillsides in the *folly, fog* and *boredom* of war.
In the Sabbath light, the hills of ink
become the torah scrolls that my son
will read from, holding the sweat
of thousands before him—All their toils
that remind us of what
is worth keeping, what we take
at a moment's notice—The hand
of a loved one, the prayers in the hills.

Disclosure

From where I stand

the stairs creak with light

replete with magic. Or mischief?—

My hands are pulled by a theatre

grassed in shepherds

       herding the lambs—

iambs, where sounds are words

holding their own. In a kitchen

ginger-bread men turn to soldiers

then drones disappearing

to the blue. I know now

that death is the sailor's grip

       corrupt and white-gloved,

climbing up the casket. On the *News*

they're dropping dainty

little bombs—or bombshells,

       little baton-twirlers

batting their eyes. Our shadows

are sweet talking in a hotel room

       on company time.

Last seen, I took off with

the bell-hop, but really

it was only a pencil, dragged heavy

       I carried it on my back.

A pink eraser, my comrade,

my lover, shavings of pink-slips,

an assembly-line of secrets.

       Off with the hooks,

heads, helmets, ailments, elephants—

The long-eared ones who promised

       never to forget. This wreckage

is a city out-lined in chalk. The walls hear

alien nation or *alienation, a nation*

of fists. This urgency of state says, *Stop here—*

You can't come—Stop here!

Beware of the lambs, thumbs

       the sheep dressed

in wolf's clothing—Even the zebras

walk off the plank two by two—

But really they are men

in pin-striped suits,

shredding the evidence

like bras of familial love.

But it's homelessness that

kills us in the end. As I pushed

the pencil, my heart was stolen

by a carpenter who wanted

      to be a surgeon from

the first time he held

the tip in his hand—Now

a woman will die of a botched

hysterectomy—Red-stained linen

      drying on the laundry line

of our grief. The shadows are

telling all. Our souls stolen

by a bloodbath of church bells,

pool halls, shopping malls—

We are all here, then we are gone.

Montage Obscura

Only your good side shows. You can jostle
a smile around the dental work
until little murmurs
heckle from hall mirrors.
                        It's always the tail-end
of summer in our backyards. Cicadas
and crickets thrum in your throat—
You could almost cough up
your heart—aching *hand-held device!*
Because the past tense lives
in strictest confidence. Slightly
out-of-focus, waiting for the explorers
to come—We're not very photogenic.
                        We heed to the infant
ones, who croon in the tiniest
of socks. Our sobbing is only
a chemical process. This is an elixir,
our secrets are kept radiant and illumined—
                        Not that they meant you
any harm, shadows folded on shadows,
an industry unto themselves.
Now juxtaposed and cross-referenced,
for *brace yourself—*
                        a kind of happiness!
It's 2011, *Lady Gaga* is a volume
balloon grandfathered in to say,
                        "We were born this way."
The clouds are brass bands. The sky
is bluer than a rumor. Your siblings will be forever
                        dripping in their swimsuits.
We were happy and wide-open
like hotels where all the people
                        have now left for home.
We were loved and gathered,
and washed away with the tide.

Your son's breath smells
of pencil erasers and lavender,
the medicine from your father's liver.
Your sister's laugh is filtered
with quivers, cropped to pierce
the heart, high in the pixilated trees.

Notes

The poem, "Hillsides" owes a great debt to this (referred to as "Hillsides") by the artist, Philip Guston, untitled, ink and acrylic, 1980 [works on paper, Morgan Library and Museum]

The poem, "Vacation" calls on and is illuminated by Martin Luther King, Jr. and his impacting "Letter From a Birmingham Jail"

"Dear Reader" owes a debt of gratitude to Italo Calvino's, *If on a Winter's Night a Traveler* (Harcourt Brace & Co. 1981)

"In Plain Sight" uses influences from Virginia Woolf's, *On Being Ill* (Hogarth Press, 1930). In 2002 Paris Press rescued and reprinted this wonderful essay

"Without A Visible Sign" takes its title from a music composition by Jan Garbarek, from *"In Praise of Dreams,"* Recorded by ECM, 2003

"Montage Obscura" uses the line, *"We were born this way,"* from Lady Gaga's song of the same title, Streamline Records, 2011 ©

Thank you to Emily Dickinson, *"Silent as a disc on a dot of snow,"* from "Letter to Metaphor"

"Frankenstein Meets Francis Bacon" owes a debt to the works of Francis Bacon, *Untitled (Three Figures)*, 1981, Dublin City, Gallery, The Hugh Lane © The Estate of Francis Bacon

Author Note

Cynthia Atkins was born and raised in Chicago, IL., receiving a BFA and an MA from the University of Illinois and an MFA from Columbia University's School of the Arts. Atkins is also the author of *Psyche's Weathers* (CW Books, 2007). Her poems have appeared in numerous journals, including, *Alaska Quarterly Review, American Letters & Commentary, BOMB, Del Sol Review, Florida Review, Harpur Palate, The Journal, North American Review, Seneca Review, Tampa Review, Valparaiso Review* and *Verse Daily,* among others. Atkins' poems were nominated for a 2011 and 2012 Pushcart Prize. Formerly, Atkins worked as Assistant Director for the Poetry Society of America. She has taught English and Creative Writing at various colleges and is currently Assistant Professor of English at Virginia Western Community College. She was founder and artistic director of Writers @ Jordan House/FAIR (reading series and workshops). She lives on the Maury River of Rockbridge County, VA with her husband, artist Phillip Welch, and their family.

CPSIA information can be obtained at www.ICGtesting.com
Printed in the USA
LVOW08s1753160114

369732LV00005B/734/P

9 781625 490339